MATING IN CAPTIVITY

7 Ways To Bring Eroticism Into Your Relationship

ELMER BRYAN

ISBN: 9781976812781

TEXT COPYRIGHT © ELMER BRYAN

TABLE OF CONTENT

INTRODUCTION

Have you ever wondered what sex is all about? We don't give much thought to sex. I mean, it is inborn, it is something we engage in as adults. We consider it one of our basic right. True? One journalist once compared music and sex. He said that the two are all about tension and release, the eagerness and restraint, the gratification and generosity, and the control and surrender. It is about delicately opposed forces in a more or less graceful fumble towards ecstasy.

Unless and until we understand the role of sex in a healthy relationship, we cannot have a healthy relationship. This EBook offers the guide on how to restore intimacy in a relationship and keep the fire burning. I will start by discussing intimacy and how to restore intimacy. It goes deeper and offers the guide to eroticism in a relationship. Lastly, the book offers a guide to having an erotic relationship, including erotic sex in which all partners enjoy orgasm.

There are times when things will not be smooth in your relationship. It is very normal. Issues arise that need to be addressed. If much attention is not given to each other, the relationship becomes flat and stale. Normally, it comes to that when the partners have conflicting attention or are distracted by other issues. In some cases, lovers have difficulty expressing what is really in their mind in a loving and caring language that their partners can understand. In most cases, intimacy is the first casualty in the case of a conflict in a relationship. It is often difficult to figure out how best to recover intimacy in a relationship.

The main goal in any intimate relationship is the feeling of a deep connection in a spiritual way between the partners. Intimacy in a relationship is associated with a safe, respectful and a supportive environment where all lovers feel wanted, appreciated, taken care of, accepted with no conditions and loved for what they are, and for the mere fact that they are alive.

But as we are going to find out, intimacy is all about being free and trusting each other. This is where Tantra sex and eroticism comes in. Enjoy!

Chapter 1: From Intimacy To Eroticism

Saving Your Relationship - Dealing With Lack Of Attraction

Saving the relationship for people who are in long-term relationships may be a problem, they are not attracted to their partners anymore, in spite of the attachment they share, the level of physical intimacy in the relationship begins to sink. Consequently, the relationship starts to feel stale. If you are in the same boat and are no longer attracted to your partner, don't think that this mindset is permanent, and neither should you be blaming yourself. You can get a positive message across to your partner and take some fruitful steps to bring the excitement back in your relationship.

Refreshing Your Partner's Memory: Think back to the time when you were attracted to your partner. What was it about them that turned you on? It may have been the looks, the laugh or the spring in their step, then the thought of saving your relationship never crossed your mind. Your relationship was blooming. Whatever it was, it is probably missing now, and you are thinking of ways and means to save your relationship. Maybe he or she doesn't spend that much time and effort trying to look attractive. What you can do is to convey the message to your partner positively and gently. If it is your girlfriend, tell her that you loved the way she used to do her hair and it would be priceless to see her that way again. Just this kind of sharing will strengthen your bond and intimacy, and it is most likely that she will cooperate.

Sharing What Turns You Off: Just like there probably are things that your partner doesn't do anymore, there may also be behavioral patterns that turn you off. Perhaps he has a very ungainly way of sitting with you at home. Once again, try to tell him gently and tactfully. Also, you need to put your criticism across positively. What you need to emphasize to your partner is what you would like about them better, rather than what you dislike about them. Polite frankness works wonders to give the right message and help you save your relationship.

Accepting Feedback: Be prepared for the fact that just as your partner is not turning you on anymore, you may not be coming across as attractive to them either. So, while you are giving inputs to your partner, encourage them to do the same as well. What you need to do is work together to bring the smile back in your relationship.

The excitement in the Bedroom: One thing that will do wonders for the relationship is if you can spice things up in the bedroom. Create the right mood for an intimate evening, and dedicate all that time with your partner. Make sure you both dress well and look pleasing, and you may just find your desire racing back, you are on the right track to save your relationship.

Improving Health: One major reason why levels of physical intimacy retard for a lot of couples is neglect to their health. The stress at work may be up, you may have put on weight, and your energy levels may have fallen. The same has probably happened to your partner. Try to incorporate some exercise into your routine. If you can do it together, that will be great to revive your bond. You both will start looking and feeling better, your hormonal balance and overall mood will improve, and your energy levels will go up. All these will impact your sex drive favorably.

With these steps, you will certainly begin to feel closer and more attracted to your partner once again, after all, you have to save your relationship that you have nurtured so intensely.

10 Step Guide To Recognize Intimacy In Relationship

You can describe an intimate relationship with the following statements:

1. It is characterized by a continuous and honest communication. This includes a constant contact with one another either directly or through other means like letters, email, phones, and text.

2. It is also characterized by the willingness to carry out mutual tasks together. Such tasks are discussed and enjoyed together.

3. It is also characterized by the affinity to one another. Such attraction and affinity to one another exist to the exclusion of others.

4. The partners always seek the company of one another, even when presented with a wide pool of other individuals and activities to choose.

5. With such lovers, there is always a sixth sense to facilitate your communication. Lovers don't need words to convey their messages to each other. Nonverbal communication is very effective in such cases.

6. There is a highly developed sense of humor and casualness between the lovers. The relationship is characterized with playfulness and give and take without resorting to intense negotiation. Lovers feel relaxed in the company of each other.

7. The relationship is also associated with high level of protection (a sense of privacy and guardedness). The lovers do their level best to protect their relationship from judgment, public scrutiny, and criticism.

8. All partners in the relationship view it as a productive enterprise that results in a mutual satisfaction, general reward for everyone and the reinforcement for each other.

9. The relationship is characterized by a sense of direction, purpose, and order. It is a reasonable and realistic engagement and is healthy for both of the partners.

10. It is also associated with the existence of unwritten but firm commitment, contract or agreement in which each other partner plays his or her role, is supportive, understanding and readily accepts the other.

Chapter 2: Intimacy, Eroticism, And Orgasm

Intimacy And Sex

For the majority of couples, the love making process is usually associated with some sense of intimacy as well as emotional closeness. For an intimate sexual relationship to occur, there is some level of trust and vulnerability between the couples. Sex also bring couples closer together, which has a profound effect on the other forms of intimacy.

With this in mind, it is important that the two partners share a whole range of emotions, failure of which one partner may feel neglected and lonely even in a relationship with many years of sexual experience. In the later topics, we discuss how a couple can share love and affection without necessarily engaging in the act of sexual intercourse. In fact, the couple that is more intimate with each other is more likely to enjoy a fulfilling sex life.

There are several barriers to a healthy sexual intimacy, some of these include:

- The fear of sex

- The impotency and ejaculation issues (lack of ejaculation or premature ejaculation)

- Sexual problems that are physically based

- Lack of honesty and openness in the relationship

- Unwillingness/Lack of motivation to get creative, imaginative and explore adventures

- Embarrassment between the partners in the sexual arena

- Misconception/discomfort with nudity

- Cultural, social, moral, and religious beliefs leading to hang up

- Unwillingness to create an encouraging environment

What is the Solution?

1. **Diagnosing the problem**: It starts with you, before blaming your partner, take some time to examine your own lifestyle to determine if you are allocating enough time for sex. You need to understand that sexuality is not an event, but it is an ongoing process.

2. The second step is to **determine why sex and intimacy dropped so low** on your priority list. Upon becoming mums and dads, most couples forget the friendship that once thrived among them. It is a big mistake to neglect your roles as lovers even after assuming the role of parenthood. If there is a problem in this area, find a way to reconnect, even if it means spending less time in the office and more time together. You must find a way of sacrificing other commitments for the sake of your relationship.

3. **Move sex to the top of the priority list**: Work together with your partner through a conscious decision to recommit in your relationship and make sure sex moves to the top of your to do list. In order to nurture physical intimacy in your relationship, you will need a lot of attention and commitment. However, it is possible to achieve this. Just start with minor changes. For example, you can resort to putting the kids to bed earlier than usual to have more time together. Don't fall asleep on the couch and try to go to bed with your partner at the same time.

4. **Make more changes**: There are always areas that you can make changes. Just take time to figure them out. Remember that men react most to the visible stimulations. Is there anything you can do in this area to stimulate him? If you are a man, keep it in mind that women are most stimulated by emotion and verbal connections. They need lots of gentle touch, hugs, and kisses. Before moving to intercourse, make sure that you spend adequate time in this areas. More of these are discussed in the next chapters.

5. **Allow yourself the freedom to have what you desire** through the willingness to claiming your rights and voicing your needs in a relationship. Remember that sexual satisfaction is a legitimate need just as the need to feel wanted by your partner.

6. **Share your concerns**: Always share with your partner about your concerns and needs. But you must be sensitive to time and place when bringing these issues up. Don't expect a good outcome if you only bring such issues in a middle of an argument. If there are other factors that might be responsible for low sex drive in your partner, you need to be supportive. The factors to look out for include medication, depression and stress among others.

7. **Stop the Complaint**: Instead of focusing on and complaining about what you are not getting, try focusing on what you really want and appreciate what you are already getting instead. It is common for women to take the marital problems so personal and end up feeling sorry for themselves. You should not assume a victim mentality but instead, focus on making changes.

8. Lastly, **work with your partner on a plan that can result to deeper intimacy**. If you share the plan, both agree on it and are excited about it; it becomes easier and exciting to put it into action. Check on chapter five about this.

Keeping Intimacy Alive

Clearly, intimacy in a relationship is a conscious choice that partners have to make on a daily basis. This is will be made clearer in the subsequent topics. With this, it is clear that intimacy is a matter that cannot be left in a corner and only attended to when partners have extra time. In healthy relationships, intimacy is characterized by a continual recommitment to a relationship and its renewal. It requires constant freshness. It is also true that intimacy is a delicate state of affairs that needs to be re-created from moment to moment in a relationship. It is good to often take time and think deeply about these issues. In this way, it helps create revelations for lovers.

Chapter 3: Nurturing Sexual Desire In Your Relationship

Building Anticipation: Why is it Important?

Anticipation is what you need to fuel the desire. Just like you anticipate social gatherings, dinner, concerts or any other thing, it is important to anticipate sex in the same way, if the marriage is to survive. Always set time for adventurous sexual experiences and savor them. In this manner, you get to establish a positive cycle of anticipation which comes with satisfaction and regularity. However, this is just one way of building anticipation.

You can also build anticipation when you think you have the freedom to make special turn-on requests. If you learn to make requests and go ahead to honor them, the outcome is intimacy and closeness translating to a better quality of sexual experience. It is very difficult to anticipate sex, especially in the case of marital sex that has turned into a mechanical routine.

3 Ways To Improve Sexual Intimacy

Happiness is the mark of emotional feelings, with such feelings, a partner gets more bonded and committed to his or her partner. This is the relational part of it. The best sex is that which is good physically, emotionally and relationally, with the third being the best. Focusing more on the most basic level (physical sex) prevents us from seeing the potential of sex beyond that basic level of it. So, the question that then follows is, why settle for only one (physical pleasure) when you can have all the three at once. Let's have a practical guide to the best sex in all the aspects.

Physically Good Sex: If you think this is the easiest to achieve and the one most of us tend to focus on the most, you are right. The next sections of the book will focus on the best foreplay maneuvers, the best positions, and secret hip movements to drive him wild and so on. These are all but physical sex information that focuses on good bedroom experiences. We may not all know it, but the best physical sex should be more about what our partner enjoys that what we enjoy. Yes, our bodies are wired differently, if you truly want to enjoy sex physically, don't waste your time on magazines, instead, find time to discuss these matters with your partner.

Emotionally Good Sex: As we have seen, sexual intimacy can be the source of much needed positive emotion. However, research has proven that not all types of sex bring the positive emotions. In some cases, it can result in negative emotions. This may be immediately after or days after the sexual encounter. Sexual encounter between people with no long term commitment or those who engage in unwanted sex are more likely to end up with depression, regret and shame instead of positive energy even if it was a willful sexual encounter. This is to say that your sexual experience should not just focus on the physical pleasure. The sexual acts should be based on mutual respect and love so that the intimacy results to positive experiences. This is to say that if you don't feel comfortable doing anything, don't force yourself expecting that in that way you will please your partner, in the same way, don't expect your partner to do anything they are not happy with.

Relationally Good Sex: When we talk of sexual intimacy, we are talking about nothing less than a bonding experience. With sex, we get bonded to one another. It does not matter if you think of sex as a spiritual encounter an evolutionary act, proper sex ends with a bonding experience. Sex offers a means to connect with your partner at the deepest possible level, this is what happens to the couples with the most satisfying sexual experience. It is important that at this stage, you re-evaluate what sex really means in your life.

Chapter 4: Erotic Talk: The Magic Of Love Making With Nothing But Words

Truth be told, for long, the role of words and verbal communication in creating fulfilling sex life has been ignored. This can be blamed on our historical perspective. In many societies, women were largely seen as sexual objects. This has, however, changed over time. So, a simple search will turn out thousands of books and articles focusing on the physical techniques that you can deploy to stimulate your spouse, the sexual position for experiencing increased passion, and the sex positions to extend the orgasms.

Sensual Talk: The Language of Love

'Talking dirty' and 'erotic talk' are two words used synonymously, but is that the case? No, that may not necessarily be the case. Well, a well-timed explicit sexual talk can offer a wonderful opportunity to enjoy the joy that comes with the intimate connection. It helps add that earthy and lusty element in love making and helps convey the intensity of your physical passion to your partner. This is what sexual experts term as the fine art of erotic talk.

However, erotic talk more complicated than a simple dirty talk. It is a communication technique that can be deployed when you are experiencing a delicate desire when feeling a very deep appreciation for your love and the pleasure your partner is bringing in, and when you are feeling playful and want to be tender. It offers a channel through which your thoughts are allowed to wander as you share sexual fantasies as well as create a dialogue that leads to enactment with your partner and lover. Erotic talk can offer an effective tool through which you can convey to your lover the awe of the depth of the spiritual and emotional connection.

You can deploy erotic talk to gather the information that you then use to arouse and satisfy your lover and also give him/her the guidance on how to please and satisfy you. If offers increased opportunities to enjoy safe and fulfilling sex. Properly deployed erotic talk helps transform the usual cumbersome and awkward love making preparation to moments of fun and exciting moments. In fact, erotic talk when well used can be a moment of lovemaking by itself. If you are figuring out how best to keep the romantic and sexual sparks alive when you are miles apart with your lover, consider the sexy communication via channels such as the emails, texts, the social media and the phone.

Love making is a connection that goes beyond the mere physical connection. It is much deeper, extending to mental connection, emotional connection, and spiritual connection as well. So, if the physical caresses and touch get us aroused and get nourished, we need their words to nourish and caress our spiritual, emotional and intellectual parts. We can reach each other's hearts and souls with the words of desire, thereby creating a profound bond that may last forever. That's how effective erotic talk can be.

So, How Do We Make Erotic Talk Part of Our Daily Life?

Imagine whispering this into the ears of your husband as he leaves for office:

> "Honey, during your coffee break, sit back at your desk, close your eyes and relax and imagine me standing behind you. Imagine my soft fingers tickling as I massage your back and neck……then the kisses follow as I unbutton your shirt….then the trouser…..honey…you can take the rest of fantasies as far as you wish…because for sure, you will have to repeat everything the first thing from work."

Nurturing An Environment For Sexual Expressiveness

An atmosphere of openness devoid of unnecessary formalities and full of play allows for the unfolding of our deepest selves and needs. The atmosphere of criticism and judgment the both in words and in the body language on the other hands causes emotional retraction. One of the most common reactions in such cases is to hide what we think is unacceptable to our partners.

Self-expression and self-retraction are two dynamic psychological events with roots deep in our childhood. As we grow up in different societies with care from different parents, we learn to react to our unfolding self-identities and needs in different ways. We learn that particular self-expressions are unacceptable and may be punishable and should, therefore, be hidden or contained to avoid the reprimand that may follow.

Chapter 5: Tantric Sex: The Secret To Eroticism

What Is Tantra?

Unknown to many of us, Tantra has been in existence for over 6,000 years. It is widely practiced in most of the eastern cultures. In western cultures and the United States, in particular, it is just being introduced. The art originates from India, where it emerged as a rebellion against organized religion. Back then, the region held that in order to reach enlightenment, sexuality had to be rejected. This was the bone of contention that gave birth to Tantra.

The acetic belief of the time held the view that sexuality was a doorway to divinity. The other popular religious beliefs were that what we now know as early pleasures like eating, dancing, and other forms of creative expressions were actually sacred acts. Tantra was challenging these religious beliefs of the time.

Tantra is a word meaning 'to show, to manifest, to weave and to expand.' In the context of sexual intimacy, sex was thought to expand consciousness as well as weave together, the male priorities (the male figure was represented by the Hindu god known as Shiva) and the female (female was embodied by the Hindu goddess known as Shakti) into one harmonious whole.

The couple that wants to benefit from this ancient art are not necessarily required to adopt the Tantric pantheon we have explained in the two preceding paragraphs. In fact, the gist of sexual Tantric practices is the art of prolonging the art of love making while utilizing the potent organic energies more efficiently.

We also benefit by learning that Tantra is also health enhancing. We don't need to overemphasize that sexual energy is ranked as one of the most powerful energy among the energies that we require for creating and sustaining good health. When used consciously, sexual energy helps us tap into the source of youthfulness and vitality.

Welcoming Love: The Core of Tantra

What kind of love making are you most familiar with? Is it often viewed as a source of reaction rather than a means of transformation? Is your goal to reach orgasm or is it to pleasure your love so that you are able to fully connect with him or her?

This is the ordinary love-making better known to the majority of us. It is associated with a distinct beginning and end. The climax often comes some in between, and the activity lasts for between 10 to 15 minutes, sometimes even less. For a woman to reach full arousal, it takes at least 20 minutes. In fact, it is often said that there are 80% chances that a woman orgasm will be realized if the sex lasts for 21 minutes. Needless to say, any sexual activity that lasts less than 15 minutes can be deeply unsatisfying.

In the Tantric model, however, a sexual act is more than just a physical and predictable activity. It is seen as a dance that has no beginning and no end. In this model, the partners are not engaging in sex for a particular goal, all that matters is the present moment of exquisite union. This means that the love making process is a meditative, expressive and an intimate process. In Tantra, the partners are taught how to extend the peak of their sexual ecstasy so that both partners are able to experience several orgasms in a single sexual encounter.

Tantra trainers help fix all bedroom issues . According to the Tantra trainers, even men that often experience premature ejaculation can be trained on how to extend their orgasm and even enjoy multiple orgasms with practice. The truth is that Tantra sex is available for all couples and partners of all ages and all levels of sexual experience. The only ingredients necessary are love, trust, and mutual respect.

Learning The Art: Tantric Intimacy Exercises

Make Time for Each Other At least Once per Week: We have already discussed the benefits of planning a sexual rendezvous as often as you can. As the first exercise under Tantra, you are encouraged to do it at least once a week, but if possible, more times. It is not as difficult as you might imagine, all you need to do is to set aside at least one hour of uninterrupted time for two of you together. Yes, I admit that in the atmosphere where we are juggling between work and home where we are overwhelmed with the children's demand for attention, it will be next to impossible to benefit from Tantra unless you maintain your relationship as number one priority.

Create an Inviting Atmosphere: It can be in the living room, verandah, bedroom, kitchen, bathroom, or any other place in your house. The place you meet does not really matter, what matters is your ability to turn that place into a sacred place. In that way, that sacred place will help you relax and bring you into the moment. How can you transform the selected room to a temple of sexual delight? This is not difficult, in fact, you don't need to overspend. Try simple things like playing with colors and smell. Use candles, fresh flowers, tantalizing aromas, finger foods and erotic art among others. You can create a welcoming environment in many different ways, including dimming lights and erotic music.

Using Ritual for Developing Intimacy: How do you begin every sexual journey with a ritual? Does it have to be a ritual of sex only? No, remember that intimacy is something beyond physical pleasure only. We already discussed the differences between the physical pleasure, the emotional pleasure, and the ultimate relational or bonding experience. This is why you need a ritual, whether before sex, when waking up or before leaving for the office. Rituals can be as simple as feeding each other a delicious food or even sharing a glass of wine in the nude. There are cases of a couple bathing together as a means to attune to each other. That sounds romantic! Well, that is what a ritual is all about.

Eye Contact and Breathing Exercise: Think of it this way, the only time we ever think of breathing is when we realize that we have difficulty in breathing. What we don't realize is that conscious breathing can, in fact, be a powerful aid in sexual growth. Conscious breathing exercises help quiet the mind which in turn helps us focus on each other.

How do you do a breathing exercise? Here is the simplest method. Sit quietly with crossed legs facing each other. Rest both of your hands on your knees with the palms facing up. Take soft but deep breaths, looking directly into your partner's eyes. In the same position, keep your eyes open, look directly into her, or his eyes keep gazing, gaze beyond the eyes into his or her soul. At first, it looks awkward, but with time, a sustained eye contact proves essential in building a lasting intimacy.

Appreciating Your Partner with Erotic Touch: If you are thinking of becoming better lovers, here is a pleasurable practice. It still requires that you maintain eye contact, but at this point, you don't have to worry about keeping the breath synchronized. Instead, take turns stimulating each other. Guide your partner to do it the way you want it done. You can actually describe him or her into doing it the way you like it.

While describing your desires, do it in an encouraging way, with a clear and loving manner of making requests. For example, you can soften your voice and whisper into the ears of your partner encouraging him or her to caress your penis or clitoris or any other erogenous zone. When doing so, you can ask them to apply more or less pressure, or maintain it there, to stroke in a particular pattern, to use the tongue, etc. Also, practice to thank your partner after the exercise and help him, or let her know using works, sounds or reactions when you are enjoying this sensual touch.

Continue with the exercise until you get comfortable with it. At this point, you can proceed to create "pleasure chest." This is to say that you can include any other things that excite both of you. This could range from things like a feather, a vibrator, soft fabric with specific colors, massage oil, and blindfold and loving notes for your partner among others. As you continue pleasuring each other, never be afraid to ask for something different. Keep it in mind that this is your moment for appreciation and experimentation and it is up to you to take responsibility for own fulfillment and for this reason, it is important that you ask what you want.

Chapter 6:   The Orgasm: The Guide Sexual Climax

The Basic Tantric Sex Techniques

All earlier chapters focus on the need to prepare for lovemaking and the fact that lovemaking is not a one-time event but a continuous activity. This is what is also emphasized in the Tantric traditions. We have already described several erotic rituals that focus on exchanging pleasures and awakening the senses. They also focus on how best to help couples communicate their deep physical and emotional needs to each other.

The phase we have discussed so far helps lovers to establish an intimate connection. As lovers transition into the sexual dimension, we need to learn how to maintain and heighten this intimate connection. The intimacy exercises are nothing more than extended foreplay used to titillate lovers for the intercourse that is to follow, but more importantly, to create an optimal condition for a Tantric sexual experience.

When an experiment with the Tantric techniques, don't waste time trying to determine if you are doing it right or wrong. Tantra has no place for good or bad, right or wrong, what matters is the ability to pleasure your partner and your own pleasure.

Your main goal when transitioning to sex is to maintain a state of sexual ecstasy for as long as you can. A Tantric love making process is not a time oriented process; it is a timeless and unstructured experience.

Maintaining a Deep Level of Intimacy: For this to work, you need to continue gazing into the eyes of your partner as he or she does the same as long as possible. Sprinkle his/her face, shoulders and neck with light kisses while whispering words of love and encouragement. Make sure that each of you feels loved and desired.

Keep it Slow: With a long but slow build, men are more able to control orgasm and helps pique women's arousal. The longer the partners linger in the energy building process, the longer the male partner will be able to resist ejaculation. During the process, make sure that all your attention is focused on your partner. If your thoughts wander by any chance, gently bring them back to the present moment. Channel all your energies and thoughts to your lover and the magic at hand.

Pay a Close Attention to Your Breathing Pattern: You must resist the urge to breathe quickly. It comes naturally, but you must learn to resist it. The reason for this is simple, panting and quick breathing creates arousal, which will speed you towards orgasm. So, what is the right breathing pattern? Try long but slow breathing from your belly so that you can exhale gradually. For better results, try matching your breathing to that of your partner. Alternatively, try an alternative breathing pattern where you inhale as your partner exhales. This is a good way of connecting the two of you as the energy moves back and forth.

Explore Your Duality by Varying Your Position: There is an extra sex pleasure that comes with different sex positions. It also balances the male and female energies. It allows lovers to release themselves from gender roles which allow them to engage in much deeper and more intimate sex. When men surrender, they are able to realize their full sexual potential. The male surrender is associated with softness, openness, gentleness, and vulnerability. In such moments, the female partner takes the role of directing and initiating the moves. Experiment with all positions, some of which will be male dominant while others female dominant. These positions should allow you the opportunity to explore your capacity to be strong, but still gentle, generous and receptive as well.

Reaping The Rewards: Multiple Orgasms For Males

At this point, we need to say that there is a difference between orgasm and ejaculation for men. The same is true is a Tantric sex guide. Ejaculation and orgasm often happen at the same time, but it is also possible for men to experience orgasm without ejaculating. The ability to control ejaculation enables Tantric lovers to capture and extend the magical energy of orgasm. The men that are able to hold back end up experiencing a series of mini-orgasms.

This should not be mistaken to mean that men should not ejaculate during Tantric sex. It is all about controlling your climax. The essence of this is to catch a wave of energy. It is like surfing the edging without having to go over. Below are the techniques that can help you stay in the wake.

Controlling the pub coccygeal (PC) muscles: These are muscles that run from the pubic bone to the tailbone. These are the ultimate sex muscles. They are the same set of muscles you will need to stop the flow of urine. You can condition them to the level where you are able to continue enjoying sex while controlling ejaculation. How can you tone the PCs muscles? Simple, you will need Kegel exercises.

The Kegel Exercise

The steps are simple. First, start by contracting your PC muscles 3 times every day squeezing 20 to 25 times every time. These are actually very simple exercises that you can do anytime anywhere. Just take care not to overdo it. Once you have conditioned for at least one month, try to extend the squeeze this time around holding each of the contraction for at least two seconds. Continue working up gradually to the point where you can squeeze for 10 seconds. With time your PCs will be in top shape, this allows you to pump them so as to ride the orgasmic wave and avoid gliding the brink sooner than you wish.

Relax: This sounds paradoxical, yet it is absolutely necessary that men stay relaxed during the state of arousal. So, what do you do should you feel the undulations of ejaculation? Simple, just take a slow, deep breath. Stop the intercourse for sometimes to allow your ejaculation to subside. While relaxing, focus on directing energy from the penis back to the rest of the body.

Talk and play with your partner. Meanwhile, use the break time to draw slow but deep breaths. This is a matter of experimenting. It helps you realize how much of the time you will need to before you catch the next wave. Remember, the time you need is just enough for the intensity to subside, but not too much time to lose your erection.

Put it All Together: Whenever you have intercourse, remember to thrust slowly. This allows your arousal to build slowly and gradually. Just before your excitement mounts to the climax, relax and take the time you need to cool down without losing the erection. While doing so, take that moment to tighten your PC muscles. Remember to take deep breaths. When ready, resume the love-making and continue generating the excitement.

When you realize it is the time, relax again, hold your PCs and remember a deep breath. When ready, continue until you near the crest. Next, open your eyes, then clamp down on the PC muscles. Take a deep breath once again and take time to enjoy an orgasm without ejaculation. It might take a bit of practice before achieving mastery.

The Ultimate Experience: Freeing Female Orgasm

Clitoral Stimulation: The majority of women requires and enjoys the stimulation of the clitoris and labia. Labia is the inner lips that surround the clitoris. The stimulation of these parts may be necessary to reach orgasm during sex. So, the key to sexual ecstasy for most women remain a prolonged but gentle clitoral touch. For a better experience, use sounds, guides and encouraging words as a guide to your lover, showing him just how to stroke you so.

The Sacred Spot: You know it as G-Spot, or mythic Graf Enberg Spot is what we also refer to as the sacred spot. This is a potent as well as a mysterious erogenous zone that is located 2 to 3 inches up the front vaginal channel. The idea is to slip in your ring finger into her vagina when she is aroused so that you brush against her inner walls with your fingertips.

The G-Spot is something the size of a pea and has a slightly rippled texture. For most women, gentle stimulation of the G-spot induces a powerful orgasm with some resulting to female ejaculation. However, it is important to be cautious to avoid over stimulating this sensitive spot.

We don't need to discuss the benefits of regular sex in any relation and even for physical wellness. It is a topic widely discussed in health journals, relationship magazines, and talk shows among others. The benefits ranges from improved immune system, better sleep, improved blood circulation and healthy heart to stress relief among others. It can be summarized 'with regular sex, you live longer.' However, sex is not just about penetration and male orgasm. In fact, as we have already seen, there is a lot to take place before penetration if a woman is to climax. No wonder you have sex toys to help you. These are adult toys that allow couples to enjoy sex in adventurous ways. This in turn benefit couples by laying a strong foundation to the relationship.

The Woman's Orgasms

This is the biggest headache that most couples have to deal with in their sexual relationship. Not many men are able to bring their women to orgasm. In fact, it is said that more than 75% of women are unable to orgasm through penetrative sex in comparison to over 90% of men who orgasm regularly through penetrative sex. What could be the problem?

We need to get the basics right. To begin, women require more stimulation to climax as compared to women. In fact, it is said that the longer the sex lasts, the more likely the woman is able to orgasm and the opposite is true. That said, how many men are able to last that long in bed? Certainly few. To make it worse, if not properly stimulated, the lady may experience pain as her organs are not properly lubricated.

Faking Orgasm

As many as 50% of women admits to having faked orgasm once in their life to avoid painful sex and embarrassing 'hard-working partner'. Funny enough, men don't even get to realize this. If you ask them, they will tell you that they don't know of any woman they have been with that ended up faking orgasm.

To avoid this frustration, partners should focus on foreplay and deploy other techniques like sex toys and oral sex that helps bring woman to climax faster. Foreplay does not have to start when in bed, in fact, it begins as soon as you wake up, continues when you are in the office and finally when back home in the evening. It is all about building anticipation. This include sharing naughty texts and calls and sharing intimacy when you get together as a couple.

But Why is this the Case?

During sex, a woman needs time for her mind to tune into the sensations of being stimulated. During masturbation, she has to spend a considerable time coming up with a fantasy that gets her mind going. Sometimes she may give up!

Before contemplating orgasm (alone or with a lover), a woman needs to feel some genital sensation in response to thinking about an erotic scenario. She feels a sense of excitement, perhaps an increase in heart-rate or breathing. When her clitoris is stimulated, she feels a slight tingling sensation. Mentally she is able to find aspects of sexual scenarios inherently erotic and appealing. If she is not 'in the mood,' then the idea of sexual activity does nothing for her and fantasies that would normally arouse her can seem quite unexciting.

A woman has to push her way towards orgasm at every stage with studied concentration. At no point is orgasm inevitable, except once it is already happening. It is difficult to imagine how female orgasm is possible while sleeping because it is such hard work even when fully awake. But also the psychological environment of dreams is not intensely focused enough to lead to orgasm.

Conclusion

Sexual phenomena (such as masturbation or gay sex) tend to be shocking and alien until we discover we enjoy them. Similarly, once we experience arousal, we see the positive (rather than the offensive) aspects of eroticism. Anyone who objects to eroticism does not understand the nature of arousal.

In this EBook, we have discussed in details the role of eroticism and Tantric sex in fostering intimacy in a relationship. It is now clearer than ever that both parties have a role to play. We have discussed in details how to communicate in love language, how to restore intimacy, the guide to Tantric sex, the male and female orgasm and the process as well as other erotic activities that partners can engage in without sex.

The target of this book is to rekindle the spark that once characterized your relationship. It is my hope that you have enjoyed every aspect of it. Please don't forget to share your feedback.

-- Elmer Bryan --